Medicine in sheep and goat

Copyright ©Pharm Haliruuk

Table of content

Chapter One
- Goat meat cure diabetes, ear disease etc

Chapter Two
- Importance of goat and sheep meat in the body

Chapter Three
- Overview of diseases and drug needs for sheep and goats.

CHAPTER ONE

Since it has become so obvious that individuals with diabetes can eat goat meat, you shouldn't get confounded and begin eating goat meat consistently. The abundance of anything is horrendous.

Diabetes patients need to control their weight, and thus, they need to keep up with their food admission. The part likewise assumes a significant part.

You ought to check how much goat meat you are consuming. Here are the different motivations behind why diabetes patients ought to consume goat meat.

Goat meat is a generally excellent wellspring of lean protein and has low cholesterol content contrasted with the different kinds of red meats.
Vitamin B12 is fundamental for the human body, and most veggie lover food things don't comprise this component. Goat meat has vitamin B12, and that is one justification for why you ought to eat it.
Goat meat additionally has more potassium and sodium, which is expected for diabetic patients.
Is goat leg soup great for diabetes?

Diabetes patients can devour any food that has goat meat in it since goat meat is sound. Goat leg soup comprises goat leg bones, spices, flavours, and different vegetables and spices.

It further develops insusceptibility and is reasonable for patients with diabetes.

Patients with diabetes shouldn't polish off sweet food sources and beverages since they are high in carbs and can expand their glucose levels.

If a diabetes patient eats such food varieties, they might become overweight and begin experiencing different sicknesses like heart illnesses or liver sicknesses.

Diabetic patients ought to follow a sound eating routine and try not to eat garbage and greasy food. In any case, what might be said about red meat? Could diabetic patients at any point consume red meat?

Assuming you have diabetes, it doesn't generally imply that you want to quit eating a wide range of non-veg food things and become a vegetarian.

Eggs comprise protein and are perfect for diabetes and can further develop blood glucose levels. You can eat chicken also. In any case, most dietitians and specialists prompt their patients not to eat red meat like hamburgers, pork, sheep, and sheep meat.

We will tell you is goat meat great for diabetes or not.

Here is the rundown of supplements that are available in goat meat.

1. Vitamin B12
2. Creatine
3. Niacin
4. Zinc
5. Iron
6. Thiamin
7. Riboflavin

Consuming red meat can be unfortunate for diabetes patients, as it has many dangers. Red meat can cause cardiovascular infections, ongoing aggravation, and different sicknesses.

However, goat meat isn't unsafe, and diabetes patients can take it in a restricted sum. Indians favour chicken over goat meat, however, they need to realize that goat meat is better and is a superior choice.

Goat is shockingly solid contrasted with the typical meats we consume, even chicken! Posted on May 6, 2012, by Suzanne Pish, Michigan State University Extension Goats are rapidly turning into a typical sight along the side of the road and on little homesteads all around the United States. Hamburger, chicken, and pork are all the more generally eaten at the American family supper table such countless individuals are astonished to discover that goat is the universe's most famous meat. Around 75% of the universe's populace eats goat meat. The interest in goat meat has risen strongly with America's developing populace of ethnic gatherings who are more acquainted with this food. American makers are battling to stay aware of the developing interest for an item that was practically incredible quite a while back. Notwithstanding the ethnic populace that routinely consumes goat meat, numerous Americans are finding the advantages of eating goats as well. Since we raise goats for meat, we frequently are inquired as to why. It tastes great and is extremely sound. It is low in fat, cholesterol, calories and immersed fat. Truth be told, goat meat is north of 50% lower in fat than our American hamburger and is around 40% lower in immersed fat than chicken - even chicken cooked with the skin off! The accompanying meat examination (per 3 oz. simmered meat) table is from the USDA: Cooking goat can be to a greater extent a test because of its low-fat substance. Cook goat meat gradually and at low temperatures to keep it from drying out which makes it extreme. The most ideal ways to cook goat are broiling or braising. Cooking should be possible in the broiler, in a smoker, or on the barbecue. Braising includes cooking it with added fluid

Goat Meat Does Not Cause Increased Blood Pressure Faculty of Agriculture, University of the Ryukyus, 1 Subaru, Nishihara-Cho, Okinawa 903-0213, Japan *Corresponding Author: K. Sunagawa. Tel: +81-98-895-8798, Fax: +81-98-895-8734, E-mail: pj.ca.uykuyr-u.rga@490689b Received 2013 Jun 7; Revised 2013 Aug 30; Accepted 2013 Aug 23. Copyright 2014 by Asian-Australasian Journal of Animal Sciences This is an Open Access article appropriated under the conditions of the Creative Commons Attribution Non-

Commercial License which grants unhindered non-commercial use, conveyance, and generation in any medium, gave the first work is appropriately referred to. While there are relentless bits of gossip that the utilization of goat meat dishes increments circulatory strain, there is no logical proof to help this. Two trials were led to explain whether pulse expansions related to the utilization of goat meat dishes. In test 1, 24 Dahl/Iwai rodents (15 weeks old, body weight 309.311.1 g) were equally isolated into 4 gatherings. The benchmark group (CP) was taken care of an eating regimen containing 20% chicken and 0.3% salt on a dry matter premise. The goat meat bunch (GM) was taken care of in an eating routine containing 20% goat meat and 0.3% salt. The goat meat/salt gathering (GS) was taken care of by an eating regimen containing 20% goat implied and 3% to 4% salt. The Okinawan mugwort (Artemisia Princeps Pampan)/salt gathering (GY) was taken care of by an eating regimen containing 20% goat meat, 3% to 4% salt and 5% of freeze-dried mugwort powder.
Examination 1 ran for a time of 14 weeks during which time the pulse of the creatures was recorded. The GS, and GY bunches polished off fundamentally more water ($p<0.01$) than the CP and GM bunches notwithstanding the way that their eating routine utilization levels were comparable. The body weight of creatures in the CP, GM, and GS gro

Medical advantages Of Goat Meat For Brain (no.21 Is Spectacular)

Home Food and Beverages Meats 28 Health Benefits of Goat Meat for Brain (No.21 is Spectacular) 28 Health Benefits of Goat Meat for Brain (No.21 is Spectacular) American and European are most popular as the universe's greatest utilization of meat yet goat meat isn't on their top rundown. Goat meat which is additionally notable as lamb or chevon is just well known in Asia. Particularly, in India however, there are a few foods produced using goat meat found on Mexican tables. The medical advantages of goat meat are likewise preferably known in Asia over in western nations. Nonetheless, don't be mixed up goat meat with sheep meat since they are very surprising creatures. In the meantime, goat meat can be handled as soup, steak, or one more cooking menu with high supplements. Why You Should Consider Consuming Goat Meat? With such a lot of fame for hamburgers, chicken and pork, why ought goat meat to become one of your choices? The issue with goat meat is, is firmly connected to certain cardiovascular circumstances particularly hypertension or the raise of the pulse. Individuals with those ailments ought to stay away from goat meat completely. Be that as it may, do a wide range of meat could cause similar circumstances whenever consumed in large part? Moreover, there are more about goat meat that you should know first and some of them are most likely the valid justifications you've been searching for why goat meat ought to be on your supper table. Goat meat is the least fatty meat. Indeed, in all honesty, yet fat contained in goat meat is lesser than the fat contained in chicken. Thus, the chicken bosom isn't the main wellspring of fatless protein for your solid way of life, goat meat could be the other option. Contrasted with hamburger, pork and chicken which were plant cultivated, goat meat was cleaner since the goat was brought up on little size ranch where the goat is meandering around eating

For the majority of diabetic patients, the objective is to keep their glucose level at the typical reach to forestall setting off other more awful difficulties that could for all time hurt their wellbeing. The most effective way to forestall glucose rise is to decrease cholesterol and sugar fixation in feasts effectively.

Likewise, a critical lessening in immersed fat is imperative. Shockingly, goat meat ticks the overwhelming majority of these containers.

With the different medical advantages related to goat meat, diabetics will handily find goat meat smart for diet consideration, and master research upholds this case. For instance, the American Diabetes of Association records lean meat as the best kind of meat to go for. Goats are perhaps of the choicest lean meat, and in that capacity, diabetics will find happiness deciding on them contrasted with other red meats.

The Food and Safety Inspection Services (FSIS) arrangement of goat meat as lean meat just affirms its agreeableness to glucose. The foundation expressed the various ways one can eat goat meat.

Diabetic patients ought to consider cooking and bubbling in low intensity rather than broiling. You can store goat meat remainders in a fridge or microwave. Nonetheless, once taken out, you ought to guarantee

you consume them in no less than 24 hours for the best advantages.
Given the advantages of goat meat, there's no question that diabetes can add it to their eating routine. Be that as it may, utilization should be moderate to try not to stuff in an excessive number of calories as you're additionally liable to get calories from other food.

Goat meat doesn't increment blood glucose levels, and it is being practical without fat makes it a favoured choice for individuals hoping to get more fit. All things considered, it's a decent expansion to a diabetic eating regimen and, when eaten respectably, can furnish an immense measure of protein with very nearly zero drawbacks.

With that far removed, it's vital to appropriately design a feast that consolidates goat meat to try not to make an unevenness. Utilizing a diabetes dinner organizer, like Klinio, can assist you with including the perfect food at the ideal opportunity to guarantee that your glucose is consistently taken care of. This virtual well-being right hand likewise a

CHAPTER TWO

A great many people believe that eating a lot of red meat is terrible for your heart's well-being over the long haul.

A rising number of specialists, in any case, are saying that goat meat has various healthful advantages. Low in calories, complete fat, immersed fat and cholesterol than conventional meats, goat meat has more elevated levels of iron when contrasted with a comparative serving size of a hamburger, pork, sheep and chicken. Nearly, goat meat likewise contains higher potassium happy with lower sodium levels. Offering more dietary benefits and more noteworthy medical advantages, goat meat has various medical advantages, which incorporate…

With regards to fat, goat meat is more slender than different meats. It likewise has far lesser calories, and that implies it is great for those attempting to adhere to an eating regimen. - While red meat is known to be high with immersed fat that increments cholesterol levels and prompts coronary illness, goat meat is said to have exceptionally low degrees of soaked fat and will represent no mischief to your heart's wellbeing. The low degrees of soaked fat in goat meat is said to further develop blood cholesterol levels and straightforwardness irritation.

- With cholesterol levels shooting through the rooftop in many families, watching your diet is significant. Goat meat involves next to no cholesterol and consequently, can be consumed consistently.

- Goat meat additionally contains more elevated levels of iron than chicken. Iron is a significant supplement, particularly for ladies — an absence of iron stores is known to cause weakness.

The meat is likewise loaded with proteins — another significant supplement the body needs consistently.

- Goat meat includes Vitamin B, which is known to assist one with successfully consuming fat. In this way, a little part of the meat is great for those needing to lose some weight.

- It is loaded with Vitamin B12, which is known to assist you with getting solid skin.

A significant number of us believe goat meat to be an uncommon delicacy that is possible at any point delighted in while feasting in a Middle Eastern or Indian eatery.

Certain individuals accept that goat meat is hard, farm meat that is in some way or another less alluring than hamburgers, pork or sheep. Well in this article we will show those individuals the method of the goat and the framework for each of the mind-boggling advantages of goat meat.

From brilliant Caribbean goat curries to Vietnamese hot wok threw goat with chillies, goat meat is a flexible red meat that conveys a superbly rich flavour.

The incredible flavour isn't the main thing that goat meat has made it work. It's additionally perfect for our planet and loaded with medical advantages.

On the off chance that you've never attempted goat or have some misgivings to try and consider goat meat as a substitution to the more normal hamburger or pork, then keep perusing to find the reason why now is the right time to put goat meat on the menu!

1. Goats are Good for our Planet

The main thing to note about goats is that they are perfect for our planet. They are one of a handful of the tamed creatures that leave the land somewhat better compared to the track down. They do this by remaining alive on the weeds and plants that different creatures disregard.

They can assume an essential part in a ranch's environment as well. For instance, whenever pigs have searched an area of forest, goats will finish and hoover up the excess brush, weeds and grass. An effective method for considering goats resembles little grass trimmers!

2. Goat Is ideal for Slow Cooking

Goat is the ideal meat for a sluggish cooker curry or stew. The gentle flavour stands up well to rich flavours like cardamom or cloves without overwhelming them. An overall extraordinary impartial meat allows the flavours to become the overwhelming focus in any dish.

To guarantee the greatest cooperation on the flavour front between the flavours and the meat, goat meat ought to be marinated for the time being. This gives the flavours additional opportunity to infiltrate profound into the meat and for a genuine profundity of flavour to be accomplished.

In the wake of marinating your meat, we figure the very best method for cooking it is using a sluggish cooker. The rich profundity of flavour obtained during the marinating system will genuinely introduce itself once the goat has been slow-cooked for about 5 hours.

It is overwhelming, dissolve-in-the-mouth meat that is, appropriately, proceeding to fill in notoriety all through the UK.

3. It's low in Fat

With regards to the numerous medical advantages of eating goat meat, how about we start with its low-fat substance.

Goat meat is less fatty than the more normal meats available like hamburgers, pork or sheep.

For each 85g serving of goat meat, there are around 122 calories and simply 2.6 grams of fat. Assuming we contrast these figures with the equivalent measured serving of hamburger, you are taking a gander at 245 calories, so over two times the sum! 85 grams of hamburger likewise has about 16 grams of fat so right multiple times the sum that of goat meat.

4. It's low in Cholesterol

Notwithstanding its low-fat substance, goat meat is additionally low in cholesterol counts.

As a matter of fact, out of Pork, Chicken, Lamb and Beef, a goat has the most reduced cholesterol counts. For each 85g of goat meat, there is around 63mg of cholesterol. Hamburger then again has around 73mg of cholesterol while chicken has 76mg per 85g serving.

Goat meat has lower by and large fat, soaked fat and cholesterol levels than other, more normal meats like Beef, Pork and Lamb. The beneath table truly places things into point of view while contrasting goat with the more famous meats in the UK.

5. Goat Is High in Protein

On the protein side of things, Goat offers around 23 grams of protein for each 85g serving.

Goat meat, in the same way as other different sorts of red meat, is a rich wellspring of protein that keeps up with strong wellbeing. It flaunts a comparable fundamental amino corrosive profile to that of chicken, meat and pork as well.

This implies that goat is all a lean meat that gives every one of the fundamental amino acids without adding any superfluous calories.

6. It's Rich in Calcium and Potassium.

Goat meat is wealthy in calcium and potassium as well.

For each 100g of goat meat, you are taking a gander at around 385mg of potassium. For a similar measure of meat, you will view it as around 316mg of potassium while chicken has quite recently 223mg.

Potassium is, obviously, incredible for keeping up with a solid pulse and for guaranteeing heart wellbeing. It manages liquid equilibrium and is one of the main minerals for the body's sensory system.

8. Elevated Degrees of Iron

The degree of iron found in goat meat bests each of the other, more normal meats we consume consistently. For around 85 grams of goat meat, you are taking a gander at 3.3mg of iron. This sum pairs chickens 1.5mg and destroys hamburgers 2.9mg.

9. Low In Sodium

At long last, Goat meat has extremely low degrees of sodium, particularly when contrasted with chicken and hamburger. The low sodium content makes goat the ideal red meat for anybody hoping to lessen their sodium utilization, however not penance on flavour or surface.

With goat meat making up more than 60% of red meat consumed around the world, it's nothing unexpected that the interest in goat meat is on the ascent here in the United States. As a country, we import more than $30 million in goat meat every year, with over a portion of that approaching from Australia. What is a shock is that it is so challenging to track down in the supermarket.

Here in the US, goat meat is undeniably more famous among workers. It's a social decision, similar to that of sheep meat. Goat meat, otherwise called chevon, is a well-known decision of meat in Mexican, Indian, Middle Eastern, Asian, African, Greek and Southern Italian foods.

Supplements in Goat Meat

The potential medical advantages of goat meat are: a rich wellspring of proteins, helps in the counteraction of cardiovascular illnesses, advances solid wellbeing with strong cell reinforcements, and has low sodium content.

Goat meat is an incredible wellspring of protein, is effectively edible, and when not corrupted with development chemicals, is a very solid lean meat. It is a hatchet phenomenal choice for hamburgers and pork, and, surprisingly, chicken. It has fewer calories, and less fat and helps lower cholesterol levels.

People with hypertension, while needing scrumptious meat, ought to consume meats with low cholesterol and low degrees of sodium to advance great heart wellbeing. Goat meat offers both of these characteristics.

Here is an examination of calories and fat in 3-ounce servings of goat, meat, and chicken:

Goat: 122 calories 2.6 grams of fat
Hamburger: 179 calories 7.9 grams of fat
Chicken: 162 calories 6.3 grams of fat
Notice the low-fat substance of goat meat. It likewise has more iron and generally a similar measure of protein contrasted with hamburgers, pork, or chicken. It is a top-notch lean protein.

Chevon gives the fundamental amino necessary acids for the general wellbeing and improvement of our bodies. It is low in cholesterol, high in protein, and a decent hotspot for individuals with a lack of iron frailty. Pregnant ladies that have low iron would likewise benefit significantly from goat meat utilization. Likewise, a decent hotspot for those who have low potassium.

Nutrients in Goat Meat

Goat meat has a variety of fundamental supplements. It has elevated degrees of Vitamin B6 and B12. Vitamin B6 plays out various capabilities in the body and is very flexible. Vitamin B12 assumes a fundamental part in the body's development of red platelets as well as keeping the sensory system working appropriately. B12 likewise assumes a significant part in our blood dissemination. Blood dissemination frees our assortments of an overabundance of homocysteine, which can cause blood clumps.

Different nutrients in goat meat are Vitamins C, E, A, and K. There are additionally micronutrients and significant minerals found in chevon that are perfect for the body: Calcium, Phosphorus, Zinc, Copper, Manganese, and Selenium.

Cooking Goat Meat

On the off chance that you're searching for a sound new protein-rich eating routine that is not white meat like chicken or turkey, goat meat ought to be first on your rundown to attempt. It's viewed as a delicacy and generally delighted in while feasting in a Middle Eastern or Indian eatery. It doesn't taste gamey and has an aftertaste like something among pork and dim meat chicken. It has a sweet, stifled flavour pr

CHAPTER THREE

Drug use in sheep

Medication is an item used to treat or forestall a sickness. Medications can assume a significant part in saving the well-being of individual sheep and the group in general. Nonetheless, they should be utilized mindfully, and makers ought to endeavour to limit drug use and not use drugs instead of good administration and taking care practices.

In the US, drugs are supported (for use) by the Food and Drug Administration (FDA). A few medications might be bought over-the-counter (OTC), without veterinary endorsement, while different medications require a veterinary remedy (Rx). OTC medications are accessible from many sources, including veterinarians, feed and homestead supply stores, and through the web. Solution (Rx) medications must be bought and utilized under the direction of an authorized veterinarian. As a rule, they should be bought from a veterinarian.

Extra-Label Drug Use

It's a given that all medications ought to be utilized as per the maker's mark or item embed. Involving a medication in any way that isn't determined on the mark requires "extra-name" drug use and should meet the necessities of extra-name drug regulations. Just authorized veterinarians might utilize or endorse sedates extra-name. Extra-name is a legitimate term. Off-name is not a lawful term. Extra-mark drugs use requires legitimate veterinarian-client-patient-relationship (VCPR). Makers shouldn't utilize sedates extra-mark, regardless of whether they can buy them OTC.

As well as utilizing a medication that isn't named for specific animal groups or classes, giving a higher dose of a "supported" drug or overseeing it alternately (SQ versus IM) additionally is extra-mark drug use. Extra-name drug use is possibly permitted when the soundness of a creature is compromised and there could be no other treatment elective. Unapproved drugs can't be utilized "off-name" to further develop execution or control generation. When contrasted with dairy cattle, ponies, and pigs, far fewer medications are endorsed by FDA for use in sheep. The Minor Use Minor Species (MUMS) regulation should make it simpler for drug organizations to get endorsements for sheep.

Withdrawal period

The withdrawal time frame is how much time it takes for a medication to "clear" the creature's framework, so that drug deposits don't stay in the tissues or milk. Each governmentally endorsed medication or creature wellbeing item has a withdrawal period imprinted on the item mark or bundle embed.

While utilized by the name, most meat withdrawal periods range from 0 to 60 days. Withdrawal periods might be different for milk and now and again, the item may not be endorsed for use in dairy females. Withdrawal periods can be a significant thought while picking which medication to use to treat a debilitated creature. Not all medications have withdrawal periods.

Withdrawal periods ought to be broadened when the medication isn't utilized as per the mark. In these circumstances or whenever a maker is dubious regarding the withdrawal time of a specific medication, a veterinarian ought to be counselled. Veterinarians approach the Food Animal Residue Avoidance Database (FARAD) which gives withdrawal data to drugs that are utilized in an extra-mark way. Extra-name withdrawal periods may likewise be accessible in logical writing.

Anti-toxins

An anti-toxin is a prescription used to treat or forestall bacterial diseases. When utilized appropriately, anti-toxins are amazing assets for keeping up with solid, useful creatures. Not all anti-infection agents work something similar and are compelling against similar microorganisms or illnesses. Here and there, lab societies are important to figure out which antibiotic(s) ought to be utilized to treat a particular illness.

Makers ought to restrict anti-infection therapy to those creatures that are debilitated or in danger of ending up being wiped out. If anti-infection agents are not utilized as expected, the chance for safe microorganisms to foster increments unnecessarily and can think twice about anti-toxin treatment. Itemized and precise records of anti-toxin medicines and results ought to be kept.

The accompanying table records the anti-microbials that are at present FDA-supported for use in sheep and sheep (in the US). The endorsed anti-microbials differ in their utilization. As of January 1, 2017, all anti-microbials considered critical to people and blended in the feed require a veterinary feed mandate (a composed request). Anti-infection agents that are placed in the drinking water presently require a veterinary solution. Aureomycin is the main anti-infection presently endorsed for use in the feed for sheep. Under the new guidelines, aureomycin might be taken care of at a pace of 80 mg for each head each day for counteraction of early termination brought about by campylobacter spp. Anti-microbials can no longer be taken care of to sheep to further develop development and feed proficiency.

An overview among little ruminant veterinary experts and makers of the United States was directed to decide the main medical conditions of sheep and goats and the requirement for medications to treat these infections. Gastrointestinal nematodes and pneumonia were the main well-being concerns. Ceftiofur, long-acting antibiotic medications, penicillins, tilmicosin and enrofloxacin were the anti-infection agents generally required. The endorsement of ivermectin and albendazole for goats, and fenbendazole for sheep were among the most well-known demands for anthelmintics. Veterinarians additionally focused on the requirement for medications to control the oestrous cycle, mitigating medications, analgesics and sedatives. Among the viral illnesses, lentivirus contaminations (ovine moderate pneumonia and caprine joint inflammation encephalitis) and sore mouth were the best worries among veterinarians and makers. The two gatherings showed that the accessibility of a conventional antiviral medication would be significant. The absence of a rabies immunization was of extraordinary concern, especially among goat makers. Extra-mark utilization of medications in food creatures might bring about drug buildups in tissues that might be unsafe for customers. Subsequently; for makers to give a superior grade, safe items while staying cutthroat in a worldwide market economy, exploration to decide security levels and tissue consumption seasons of new medications is an earnest requirement for the sheep and goat industry.

Sheep and goats, altogether alluded to as little ruminants, are a significant wellspring of meat, milk, and fleece for individuals all through the world. Gastrointestinal nematode parasites, generally called roundworms, can cause difficult sickness in these creatures. Sadly, roundworms in little ruminants are progressively becoming impervious to antiparasitic drugs around the world. The U.S. is no special case.

With the endorsement of ivermectin in 1984[1] and other macrocyclic lactones before very long, U.S. veterinarians and little ruminant makers had the option to effectively, inexpensively, and securely treat whole gatherings of sheep and goats for parasites with high introductory viability. Consolidating exceptionally viable antiparasitic drugs with the act of at the same time treating all creatures in a group or crowd — a training still normal today — can result, from the start, in a very nearly 100% parasite kill rate. Yet, ongoing logical proof shows that killing all parasites from a group or crowd isn't manageable because of the inescapable improvement of antiparasitic resistance.[2]

Antiparasitic obstruction is the hereditary capacity of parasites to endure treatment with an antiparasitic drug that was by and large compelling against those parasites before. After a creature is treated with an antiparasitic drug, the helpless parasites bite the dust and the safe parasites make due to give opposition qualities to their posterity. Broad antiparasitic opposition compromises the well-being of little ruminants and can bring about creation misfortunes for makers.

Since generally few antiparasitic drugs are FDA-supported for little ruminants, veterinarians frequently use antiparasitic drugs endorsed for different species in sheep and goats in an extra-mark way. The Animal Medicinal Drug Use Clarification Act of 1994 changed the Federal Food, Drug, and Cosmetic (FD&C) Act to permit veterinarians to legitimately endorse, under indicated conditions, a supported human or creature drug for utilization that isn't recorded on the medication's marking (this is cancelled an extra-or name use). To recommend medication in an extra-mark way, the veterinarian should follow FDA's prerequisites for extra-name drug use in creatures, as expressed in the FD&C Act and FDA guidelines.

A few antiparasitic drugs are endorsed for just sheep, so veterinarians frequently recommend these medications for goats in an extra-mark way. Because of contrasts in drug retention and digestion among sheep and goats, veterinarians generally utilize a portion in goats that is 1.5 to twice the endorsed sheep portion. Since the compelling portion in goats is presently obscure, veterinarians might be under-or over-dosing creatures, which might add to the advancement of antiparasitic opposition.

While involving a medication in an extra-mark way in food-creating creatures, for example, little ruminants, the endorsing veterinarian is liable for laying out a significantly broadened withdrawal period upheld by proper logical data.

www.ingramcontent.com/pod-product-compliance
Lightning Source LLC
Chambersburg PA
CBHW050327220526
45465CB00005B/2167